curing collagen:
forget the role of collagen for proper health and long life

By

Ann W. Peterson

Disclaimer

The information provided in this book is intended for educational and informational purposes only. It is not a substitute for professional medical advice, diagnosis, or treatment.

The authors and publisher of this book make no representations or warranties of any kind, express or implied, about the completeness, accuracy, reliability, suitability, or availability with respect to the book or the information contained in it for any purpose. You should always seek the advice of a qualified healthcare provider with any questions you may have regarding a medical condition.

Table of contents

Introduction

Amino acids make up the protein particle that form collagen. It gives connective matter extracellular space structural assist. It is the ideal matrix for skin, tendons, bones, and ligaments because of its stiffness and resistance to stretching it is good for taking care of your skin, eat a lot of food that contain collagen

Chapter 1

Definition of collagen

About 30% of its total protein comes from it. The main component of your body's skin, muscles, bones, tendons, ligaments, and other connective tissues is collagen. Your organs, blood vessels, and gut lining all contain it.

Amino acids are used to create proteins. Proline, glycine, and hydroxyproline are the three major amino acids used to produce collagen. In a triple helix configuration, these amino acids band together to form protein fibrils. To create the triple helix, your body also needs the right amounts of vitamin C, zinc, copper, and manganese.

What is collagen used for?

The major function of collagen is to give your body structure, strength, and support.

The specific roles of collagen include:

1 promoting the formation of fibroblasts, which support the growth of new cells, in your dermis (middle skin layer)2 Participating in the replacement of dead skin cells.

3 Giving organs a covering that protects them.

4 giving your skin suppleness, structure, and strength.

promoting blood clotting

Chapter 2

kind of college

There are about 28 different kinds of collagen. They vary in the way the molecules are put together, the cell part that are added, and the locations in which the body uses the collagen. There is at least one triple helix structure in every collagen fibril.

The primary five forms of collagen and their functions are:

Type 1
The most prevalent kind of collagen present in the body naturally is type I collagen. It is located in the dermis, just below the skin's surface, and makes up 90% of the body's collagen reserves. Due to its many likely lead, type I collagen can be found in most supplement varieties.

Omega-2 Collagen

Type I collagen is found in supplements made from bovine, fish, or eggshell membranes. More unbiased research is needed because many studies pointing to the advantages of these items are supported by the industry; yet, customer interest in potential support for the health of joints, hair, nails, skin, ligaments, and cartilage is significant.

Nearly 30% of the body's total protein mass and 60% of cartilage are composed of collagen.At age 30, the body's collagen production slows and starts to decline, leaving behind skin that is thinner, drier, and less elastic. Though further research is required, using collagen supplements might help reduce the impacts of collagen loss depending on your desired goal.

Before using supplements containing type II collagen, people with allergies to fish or chicken should speak with their doctor.

Although there is little current research on the effectiveness of type II collagen, preliminary studies on individuals with knee osteoarthritis found encouraging levels of pain reduction with the use of type II collagen and acetaminophen.
Omega-2 Collagen
Less firmly packed than type 11

Type ll
compared to type I collagen, collagen is less densely packed. This might mean that collagen in this form is easier for the body to digest and absorb. Increases in range of motion, a healthy reaction to joint inflammation, and the repair of worn-out joint cartilage are further potential advantages.

Collagen Type III

The second most typical form of collagen found naturaType III collagen is assumed to support the uterus, muscles, blood vessels, and stomach alongside type I collagen. The most prevalent source of type III collagen is bovine products.Although some studies suggest the body may employ type III collagen to assist combat inflammatory disorders, the body will use amino acids in any way it requires, calling into question the role supplements may play in this process. It may not always be successful to use a certain collagen supplement to target a particular section of the body.

Collagen of type V

Type V: Collagen, which is naturally present in the eye and aids in the cornea's ability to transmit light, The framework for the body's tissues and organs is built naturally by this type of collagen in together with types I and III. It is also confess that type V collagen

help the liver, lungs, muscles, bones, and cartilage
More research is required to discover whether type V collagen supplements can be metabolized by the body and used to support these areas, despite the fact that scientists are familiar with how the body utilizes its natural supplies of type V collagen. Promising study on type V collagen supplements points to potential advantages for cell membranes, the tissue in the placenta, and eye health.

Collagen of type X

Joint cartilage contains type X collagen, which is naturally present in the body and is in charge of forming bones. There is no concrete proof that taking type X collagen supplements will enable the body to directly mend an injured area.

Identification of underlying rheumatological illnesses may be aided by naturally existing type X. Specifically, those with a high level of typeharming cartilage and bone.
Type X collagen may be utilized to speed up the healing process after limb injuries and fractured

bones, according to claims made by collagen supplement firms. There is no evidence for this assertion at this time.

Chapter 3

What disintegrates collagen

Have you ever questioned why certain individuals seem to be impervious to the ravages of aging? One of the most crucial elements that can help is adequate collagen production. Let's find out more about the benefits of collagen.

You've probably seen advertisements for foods, skin products, pills, or powders that contain collagen. Collagen is an essential part of the skin that makes it flexible and strong enough to allow for mobility. The skin can create more collagen, which makes it stronger and more appealing. However, a person's lifestyle can affect how much collagen is made and how much collagen is present overall in the skin.

What, however, can harm collagen production? The precise causes change depending on the patient, what they eat, how much sun they get, and other natural causes. These dangers increase the amount of collagen that the body breaks down, causing wrinkles and drooping skin to emerge.

Collagen's Role in Skin Aging

The epidermis, dermis, and subcutaneous tissue comprise the three primary layers of the skin (fat).

1 The skin's tough outer layer, or epidermis, is where new skin cells are produced. Our skin pigment is produced in this layer, which also serves as a barrier between the body and the outside world. The five layers that make up the epidermis continuously produce new cells to replace older, dead surface cells that are constantly lost.
The skin served as the epidermis, dermis, and subcutaneous tissue are the three primary layers (fat).

The skin's strong outer layer, the epidermis, produces new skin cells. Our skin pigment is produced in this layer, which also serves as a barrier between the body and the outside world. The five layers that make up the epidermis continuously produce new cells to replace older, dead surface cells that are constantly lost.

The middle layer, known as the dermis, is composed of fibroblasts, collagen, and elastin fibers. The skin benefits from this by receiving nutrients, physical support, strength, structure, moisture, and flexibility. The dermis layer also houses lymphatic veins, apocrine glands, sweat glands, sebaceous glands, and hair follicles.blood vessels, too. The dermis' capacity to stretch and contract is due to the arrangement of collagen and elastin in its dense, woven fibers. Collagen proteins make up about 70% of the dermis. Proteolytic enzymes break down collagen fibers, which are constantly being replaced by new collagen fibers.

The skin is connected to the underlying bone and muscle through subcutaneous tissue (fat). It is a layer of connective tissue and adipose tissue (fat) that serves as insulation and cushioning for the dermis and epidermis in addition to being primarily used for fat storage.

4 **The impact of aging on skin**: The body's capacity to naturally renew collagen declines about 1.5% annually as we get older. As a result of the residual collagen strands stiffen and fray, while the elastin fibers thicken and fray as well. This

degeneration affects the structure, elasticity, and firmness of the skin, giving it an aged and wrinkled appearance.

Chapter. 4

10 indicators that you lack collagen

The best common protein in the body is collagen. Symptoms of a collagen deficit might include wrinkles, weak bones, thinning hair, and even depression.

Here, we examine various indications of collagen inadequacy as well as the most prevalent illnesses it causes:

1 wrinkle

3 Blood Pressure Levels

3 Aching Muscles

4 joint pain

6 Mobility Loss

Seven dull or thin hair

8 Dental Concerns

9 Facial Harassment

10 Leaky Gut

Wrinkles

Your skin's strength and structure come from collagen. Your collagen reserves gradually diminish as you age. Your skin starts to lose part of its structural integrity as a result, which causes wrinkles to appear, especially on the face. If steps are not done to stop this process, wrinkles will swiftly develop all over the body, causing the skin to sag.

Vital signs

Unusual blood pressure results from collagen weakness. Collagen makes up the walls of your blood arteries, and as you get older, your body has a harder time efficiently controlling blood flow since your body's natural collagen production declines. As a result, you might experience issues like chest pain, exhaustion, persistent headaches, and vertigo that are related to elevated blood pressure. Lowered collagen levels can significantly lower your quality of life. According to studies, collagen deficiency frequently goes hand in hand with low blood pressure.

Knee Pain

Your joints' cartilage is a thin tissue. Collagen is important for joint movement and function since it is a component of cartilage. Your joints' stability and integrity will deteriorate if you don't have enough collagen in your body. As a result, you can start to feel too much friction, which could eventually lead to arthritis. Joint pain can also be brought on by a lack of certain critical nutrients that are either directly or indirectly linked to the body's insufficient collagen supply. It is advised to take a high-quality collagen supplement in addition to your diet to help avoid joint discomfort and any development of arthritis.

Muscle pain

Muscles are joined to ligaments and bones by collagen. Collagen fibers become brittle due to a lack of collagen, andbones. Lack of collagen weakens collagen fibers and the connections between muscles. Your muscles start to hurt more, and there is increased friction as a result.

Chapter 5

foods to eat to increase collagen

1. Bone bouillon

Despite new research advise that bone broth may not be a reliable source of collagen, this choice is unquestionably the most well-liked among consumers. This method, which require boiling animal bones in water, is said to draw collagen. Use spices to flavor the broth while doing this at home.

Bone broth contains calcium, magnesium, phosphorus, collagen, glucosamine, chondroitin, amino acids, and many other minerals because it is comprised of bones and connective tissue,

The quality of the bones and other materials used, she continues, "make each bone broth unique.

Try preparing your own broth with bones bought from a reliable local butcher to ensure the quality of your food.

2 **Chicken**

There is a reason why chicken is used to make a lot of collagen supplements. There are many of it in everyone's favorite white meat. (You probably realized how much connective tissue poultry contains if you've ever sliced up a whole chicken.) Because of these tissues, chicken is a great food source for collagen.

3 **Marine organisms**

According to some research marine collagen is one of the uncomplicated to absorb.

despite the fact that eating salmon for dinner or a tuna sandwich for lunch can grow your collagen gain, you should be aware that the "flesh" of fish contains less collagen than other, less appetizing components.

we don't usually eat the part of fish that are highest in collagen, like the head, scales, or eyeballs." Fish skin has truly been employed by researchers as a source for collagen peptides.

4 **Four egg whites**

Despite the fact that eggs lack connective structures like many other animal products, they do contain a lot of proline.

Unreliable Source, an amino acid crucial for the formation of collagen.

5 orange fruits
The body's natural precursor to collagen, pro-collagen, is produced in large part by vitamin C. Therefore, it's important to get adequate vitamin C.

Citrus fruits including oranges, grapefruit, lemons, and limes are rich in this vitamin, as you are surely aware. For breakfast, try a grilled grapefruit or toss some orange segments into your salad.

6 berries
in spite of the fact that citrus fruits usually receive the most attention for their high vitamin C content, berries are also a great source. A berries mostly contain more vitamin C than oranges. Blackberries, blueberries, and raspberries also gives a sizable dosage.

Furthermore, berries are rich in antioxidants, which shield the skin from harm.

7 Tropical fruits:

Completing the list of wealthy fruits isTropical fruits including mango, kiwi, pineapple, and guava are high in vitamin C. A little amount of zinc, another essential for collagen formation, is also present in guava.

8 garlic

You may get more from garlic than flavor in your pasta and stir-fries. It may grow the number of collagen you make. "Garlic is high in sulfur, a mineral that support in the combination of collagen and prevents its breakdown," l

But it's determined to remember that how much you eat counts., "You surely need a lot of it to get the collagen result.

But with all of its improvement , you should think about adding garlic in your daily diet. If you love garlic, twice the amount specified in a recipe, as is advised online.

9 savoy cabbages

We all know that leafy greens are necessary to a balanced diet. It turns out that they might also give aesthetic gain.

The chlorophyll that gives salad greens like spinach, kale, Swiss chard, and others their color is recognized for its antioxidant effects.

According to certain research, eating chlorophyll causes the precursor of collagen in the skin to rise, explains Gabriel.

10 Beans

Beans are a high-protein diet that frequently include the amino acids required for the production of collagen. Additionally, a lot of them are high in copper, another nutrient required for the formation of collagen.

10 **ten cashews**

Make cashews your first option of snacking nuts the next time you grab a handful. These filling nuts provide zinc and copper, which help the body produce more create collagen

12 **Tomatillo**

One medium tomato can give up to roughly 30% of this crucial component for collagen, making it another untapped source of vitamin C. Large quantities of lycopene, a potent antioxidant for skin support, are also present in tomatoes. dependable source

13 **peppers, bell**

Add some red bell peppers to a salad or sandwich along with the tomatoes. These vegetables include capsaicin, an anti-inflammatory chemical, and are strong in vitamin C. Trusted Source that may fight aging-related symptoms.